CHIC MINIMALISM

21 RULES FOR MASTERING THE ART OF LESS

MICHELE CONNOLLY

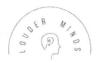

CONTENTS

Bonjour   1

01 Start From Your Values   3

02 Keep Your Sparkle - Or Your Stuff   7

03 Make Pleasure Your Guide   9

04 Let The Space Call The Shots   13

05 Know You'll Get It Wrong - And Survive   17

06 Trade Off Convenience For Simplicity   21

07 Choose Less But Luxe   25

08 Live Life As A Special Occasion   27

09 Favor Style Over Fashion   31

10 Release Gifts And Mementoes   33

11 Decide To Do Without   35

12 Don't Be A Squirrel   39

13 Discard Imperfectly   43

14 Design A Plan   47

15 Use These Three Steps Every Time   51

16 Have a Place For Everything   55

17 Break Up With Your Mess For Good   57

18 Say No - Elegance Is Refusal   61

19 Cultivate A Donation Habit   65

20 Don't Resist Temptation   67

21 Shop Strategically   69

Merci   73

About the Author   75

Also by Michele Connolly   77

BONJOUR

*W*elcome to *Chic Minimalism: 21 Rules For Mastering The Art Of Less.* In this petite guide, sophistication and simplicity don't just meet - they fall in love.

I used to feel overwhelmed by stuff, other people's expectations, and the pressure to strive for more. More possessions, achievements... everything. I could be assertive, as long as no one could hear me. Then I learned the secret to a richer life had been hiding in the negative space all along. That's what I'd like to share with you - how I came to love less and found true opulence in omission.

Do you picture minimalism as a tundra of empty rooms and unadorned walls, the dreary lifestyle of someone you might tune out at a dinner party? Then allow me to introduce its cooler cousin. *Chic minimalism* is not about stripping down to a bleak existence; it's about curating a life filled with ease, elegance, and, *mais oui*, a dash of indulgence.

In these pages, you'll discover the allure of chic minimalism: more joy, more peace, more time to savor the delicious moments life serves up - moments we miss when we're forever losing things in the morass of our homes or trying to remember the color of our countertops.

With a sprinkle of style, a soupçon of lazy, and a hint of French inspiration, I'll reveal my shortcuts to help you live with less, without losing your sparkle. I'll share ideas to lubricate our minds so things slide more easily out of our lives. Strategies for clearing the clutter jungle with a scythe rather than a Swiss Army Knife. Habits to help you finally break up with the chaos - and not let it talk its way back. Although these are rules, they are *your* rules, to embrace if appropriate and apply as you wish.

And in true minimalist style, I'll pare it all down to the essentials - no fluff, no clutter.

So, pour yourself something delightful, settle into your most comfortable chair (just move aside yesterday's outfits), and come with me on a journey that will not only declutter your space but also lighten your soul.

Chic Minimalism isn't merely a book, it's a movement - a graceful waltz away from excess, and a twirl towards things that truly matter. Are you ready to dance?

01 START FROM YOUR VALUES

*M*inimalism, having 'less', is not standard. For one person it's paring down to 100 possessions, for another it's going an entire day without screaming obscenities into the void after stepping on Lego. We're all different, and what gives us a sense of meaning and order is unique.

So the starting point for embracing minimalism is to think about what matters to you - your values. It's the foundation of all your choices and stops you getting overwhelmed with decision fatigue. *Do I keep this marble sculpture of a naked mole rat or not? HOW DO I KNOW?*

Your values help you distinguish what to keep and what to jettison, as well as what to buy and what to decline. Any other approach is guesswork. Or worse, dancing to someone else's tune - which is fine if it's an 80s classic, but other people may not have such good taste.

So then, what are your core values? Can you identify three or four of your top priorities in life? Do you most cherish family? Beautiful surroundings? Health? Hospitality? Art? Serenity? Excitement? Novelty? Education? Quirkiness? Food and cooking? Freedom? Fun?

Here are two ways to gain clarity.

1. Review lists of values.

There are plenty of values lists and quizzes online - peruse a few for the values that most resonate with you and apply to your space.

2. Consider what detectives would deduce.

You know when cops go to a murdered person's home in detective shows? They glean clues because the surroundings reflect who the person was and what they cared about, before getting savaged by the local serial killer. What does your home reveal about you? Is this accurate, or could you be a better set director for your life?

I value beauty, order, and freedom, so for me minimalism means having a few lovely things, all of them beautifully organized, with the least amount of maintenance and upkeep. More pleasure, more time.

If you prize quirkiness then that's a *yes* on the naked mole rat. If family, fun, and hospitality are key, then minimalism may mean paring possessions down by 10 or 20%, to achieve a less stressful level of joyful chaos.

Once you identify your values you can align your home to reflect them, and eliminate things that detract from your top priorities.

02 KEEP YOUR SPARKLE - OR YOUR STUFF

I struggled for years before I discovered chic minimalism. How could I feel so overwhelmed when I'd tried everything, from pretending I didn't care to procrastinating because perfectionism immobilized me?

It's not that I had a colossal amount of stuff, but I had too much *for me*. All the clothes and stationery and entertaining paraphernalia did not make me happy. The constant chaos of feeling crowded and disorganized, the frustration of being unable to find things fast, the irritation of untidiness - it left me miserable, and a little insane.

Eventually, I realized something: It wasn't possible to keep the things *and also* be happy and my most delightful self. I had to deal with my old denial and perfectionism, or accept the constant low-level discontent, knowing there was a happier way to live. I had to make a choice.

And so do you.

You have your own level of 'enough'. You cannot keep too much clutter, continue to live with mess, tolerate chaos, and also feel chic and charming. The cost is your joy, peace, calm, elegance. Your sparkle!

I won't tell you to get rid of excess, whatever excess feels like to you, or guilt you into anything. Keep the stuff if you like - most people do, after all - but recognize the cost.

Or... choose your sparkle, happiness, freedom - and, as you read on, mentally prepare to let go.

Life is already many days in a row of having to be grown-ups - let's not make it harder by adding the stress and overwhelm of too much stuff.

Before we proceed, consider these questions. Write about them or talk with a friend.

- What is clutter costing you? Time? Energy? Peace of mind? Happiness? Calm relationships? Your most chic self? What else?
- If you were to let go of some things, how would your life be different?
- How would you feel about yourself if you did that?
- Are you prepared to sacrifice possessions for happiness?

03 MAKE PLEASURE YOUR GUIDE

*P*erhaps you fantasize about your ideal home: calm, ordered, beautiful. Yes, imaginary houses are so easy to maintain. Real life has other ideas.

Decluttering can feel like drudgery - having to go through your stuff, onerous decisions about how to dispose of it, forcing yourself to get rid of things you love.

But with chic minimalism we make pleasure our guide.

1. Pleasure is *why* we choose less.

Consider some delights of chic minimalism...

- A home that feels spacious and ordered.
- The joy of being surrounded only by things you love.

- A closet that doesn't have to be wrangled like a hungry alligator for something to wear.
- Serene confidence, because you know where things are, locate them in an instant, and never fly into a panic if someone drops by unexpectedly.
- The luxury of less - less to clean, tidy, store, insure.
- The gift of time to relish life's small pleasures without the burden of perpetual reorganizing, searching, and the feeling of running in circles.
- The freedom that comes from shedding the weight of excess belongings.

2. Pleasure is *how* we choose less.

As chic minimalists, we let pleasure guide our decisions.

For example, e-readers are a fantastic way to cut down on physical books - not to mention bookshelves. But if you, like me, adore the smell of books, the tactile pleasure of holding one as you read in bed, the delight of scanning spines on a neatly curated bookcase, then keep your books!

Plus, tuning in to what actually gives you joy helps you to want less and avoid the desperate consumption that can arise when we feel unsatisfied in life.

Chic minimalism is not about deprivation - it's about having more mental and physical room to enjoy life's pleasures. Use pleasure to decide what matters to you, what is worth the space it takes up in your home and heart.

04 LET THE SPACE CALL THE SHOTS

'*Space: the final frontier*.' If even future Star Trek civilizations find 'space' an issue, how should we 21st century chic minimalists best deal with clutter?

One option is to **start with your things** and fit them into your home. This may require shelving, furniture, containers, storage cubes, shoe racks, hooks, vacuum bags, boxes. And labels! Diligent organizers do a lot of labeling. As you buy more, you need more storage. Ongoing thought, shopping, and labelling.

Instead, consider the chic minimalism approach, where you **start with the available space.** What possessions will your space elegantly accommodate? That's how many possessions you can have. No overfilling, no additional storage.

Here are some ways I've done this.

1. Hangers.

After my minimalism-inspired declutter, I bought enough lovely new hangers for my clothes - and I never buy more. My periodic closet clean-outs free up hangers, and I buy a few pieces now and then, using them up again. But I never have more clothes than hangers.

2. Closet space.

A few years ago I found myself with reduced built-in closet room. (I have a lot of outfits for someone who rarely leaves the house.) I could have bought furniture, but instead chose to let the space call the shots, and pared down my clothes. You know what? Not only do I miss nothing I gave away, I now love having less and the ease of putting together looks.

3. Makeup purse.

I have a gorgeous, tiny Saint Laurent cosmetic pouch that fits a lipstick, tiny hand cream, nail file, mini Opium spray, lip balm, and Tic Tacs. It never needs cleaning out because I couldn't get anything else in there if I wanted to. Which I don't.

4. Books.

I have a bookcase in the living room, a small bookshelf in my studio, and a shelf under my bedside chest. All my books have to fit in one of these places - and neatly! I'm always buying new titles so there's a constant stream bound for the thrift store or library.

5. Apartment.

Because my apartment is petite, I have few, compact furniture pieces. And only as many possessions as fit elegantly into the cabinets, closets, and drawers. Small spaces are the bossiest!

Let your space limit what you have. Don't buy extra storage. Avoid shunting things to the basement - save that for your handcuffs.

05 KNOW YOU'LL GET IT WRONG
- AND SURVIVE

*M*any people hold on to clutter out of fear.

What if I surrender the elliptical trainer used exclusively for clothes drapery since 2017, then feel suddenly compelled to perform simulated running with exaggerated arm gestures?

What if I rid the kitchen of myriad rarely used appliances, then can no longer channel Nigella Lawson and cook elaborate dishes while making delightful sexual innuendos?

During my major declutter many years ago I longed to be rid of things I seldom used, but I got anxious - wouldn't I need these things one day? Shouldn't I keep them, just in case?

Then I had a ~~third glass of red~~ little epiphany.

Of course I'd need some of these things. Definitely. That bizarre wooden egg gift. The leather sofa cleaning kit I bought when I forgot I am intrinsically lazy and will never clean the sofa. Or whatever. But I figured there would only be a few things I'd miss. And that realization made the choice easier.

Would I rather keep *all* this stuff for the smattering of items I might want again, or simply buy those items as needed? Or - and a shocking thought entered my mind - could I do without them altogether?

I realized with a start I could replace things I needed in the future. I could handle not owning a specific wine glass for every red varietal and yet somehow find the strength to go on.

If, like me, you've sacrificed happiness and equanimity in the present in order to anticipate every future contingency, maybe it's time to unclench. Would you rather pay for storage - in physical, spatial terms and also the psychological space our things take up in our minds - or pay for occasional replacements?

We may amass things as a security blanket, a grasp for comfort in a chaotic world. With chic minimalism you cede some choice and convenience - but unless you're a Scout you can be happily unprepared for many things. Doing without starts to become empowering, as you replace *just in case* with *I'll handle it.*

Having chosen to let it all go years ago, I can

report from the other side. There will be times you wish you still had something, but they will be rare. For the vast majority of your discarded items, you'll never give them another thought, except to notice how happy you are to be rid of it all.

I've come to enjoy the freedom of doing without something. And I love the sparse shelves where all the wine glasses used to be.

06 TRADE OFF CONVENIENCE FOR SIMPLICITY

When you possess fewer things, you surrender the illusion of control, the convenience of everything you may possibly need. But you gain the simplicity of less stuff, more space, better organized shelves, neater drawers, and greater mental clarity.

Here are some ways to make the swap.

1. Edit your closet.

Be like the French - mix and match your best pieces more often and ditch items you infrequently wear. Yes, you waive a wardrobe crammed with options - but let's be honest, most of us look and feel best in a capsule version of our clothes. And we get overwhelmed by too much choice. So this is less of a sacrifice than it appears.

2. Simplify your makeup routine.

Have you seen those celebrity videos where a 'quick' makeup uses 17 products, and wondered how they ever leave the house with the regular version? Streamlined makeup means speedy application. And more space in your bathroom cabinets and makeup purse. And my favorite, less difference between your *ooh la la* and *au naturel* faces. What could be worse* than looking so stunning when dolled up that your naked visage in the morning gives you a fright? This trade-off is easy for me because I'm essentially lazy and never learned proper makeup application skills. If you do have skills, use them to design a minimalist *maquillage*, and let the rest go.

3. Streamline recipes.

Identify the dishes you most enjoy and eliminate appliances, utensils, cookbooks, and ingredients for recipes you rarely prepare. Having a gorgeously streamlined kitchen might even make cookery more fun.

4. Cull subscriptions.

Cancel streaming services, monthly deliveries, app subscriptions - anything not worth the expense, clutter, or complication. When you need something, enjoy getting it for yourself.

5. Pare down commitments.

Withdraw from engagements that don't fit your current values and gain time, mental space, and peace of mind. If, like me, you're a hermit - I mean introvert - you probably already do this one.

Now, do I need four harps or five?

* Running out of wine would be worse.

07 CHOOSE LESS BUT LUXE

*Y*ears ago, because of circumstances well within my control, my life became chaotic - a student film with a Yoko Ono soundtrack. Too many commitments to ever truly relax. Too crowded a closet for outfit choices, making me late for everything, a trail of jilted garments in my wake.

What ignited my passion for minimalism was pivoting from *less,* to *less but luxe*. I realized that buying as little as possible meant I could afford excellent quality. This was not lack, but indulgence and thoughtful self-care.

Here are some of my favorite benefits of less but luxe.

1. Less stress.

Cheaper items invariably frustrate. Zips catch.

Designs look tacky. Legs wobble (not yours - put that cocktail down!). It all feels icky. Spare yourself.

2. More time and money.

When shoddy things inevitably break or we give up on them, there's disposal and searching and re-purchase. Quality lasts longer, needs infrequent repair or replacement, and saves time, hassle, and money in the long run. In my experience, fewer, more expensive things have cost far less than having more of the mediocre.

3. Less consumption, more space.

Have you noticed when you buy quality, you need less? One or two beautiful lipsticks rather than a drawer full of dross. A gorgeous coat that goes with everything. Select ornaments reflecting your style instead of a profusion of knick-knacks that make your eyes want to go and lie down. Less clutter and a clearer mind.

4. Planet love.

When we discard the cheap stuff, we add to landfill. The less we buy and the longer we keep it, the better for our Earth.

5. Greater pleasure.

Best of all, fewer, better things give us far more pleasure. They're a joy to use, to wear, to look at. They feel like enough, so we need little and can enjoy the added delight of aesthetically arranged shelves, tidy drawers, and unobstructed surfaces.

08 LIVE LIFE AS A SPECIAL OCCASION

One way I used to excel at life was to (1) acquire things that gave me pleasure and (2) never ever use them. I didn't believe I should enjoy myself, I was waiting for someone to give me permission. Once I realized I needed no justification for eating a Nutella cronut in the middle of a Tuesday, my real life began.

Do you save things for a 'special occasion'? But life is a special occasion! We only get one. Chic minimalists enjoy our lives now. For example...

1. Bed linen.

I have only two sets of sheets - white, high-thread-count, costly - that not only look gorgeous, but *sound* sexily swishy. They last forever, and on the rare occasion a sheet has torn, the manufacturer replaced it.

2. Towels.

My two sets of luxurious bath towels dry fast and feel super fluffy. Their charcoal color looks great against white tiles and matches my home decor.

3. Tableware.

Instead of *everyday* versus *guest* plates, glassware, and napery, I have great quality items that get used whether it's pizza on the sofa or a dinner party (don't worry - I order in). They come in singles for replacing breakages.

4. Perfume

I wear *parfum* every day - even if it's only me at the keyboard in activewear, or on the sofa with pizza (hmmm, this comes up a lot). French houses like Chanel take scent seriously, but I also like heady throwback fragrances like Obsession and Aromatics Elixir. Wear what you love.

5. Skincare and makeup

I enjoy using only the basics in skincare and makeup - which means I can afford excellent products. If in doubt ask your dermatologist, who'll tell you to avoid pseudoscientific potions making outlandish claims. Except for active water channeling age reversal from the moon - that stuff *works*.

6. Journals and pens

If a notebook had a pretty cover, I coveted it. But many have cheap paper and yucky line spacing. Now I use Moleskine and LEUCHTTURM1917 journals, and a white and rose gold Montblanc fountain pen to write in them. Using the 'best' (for me) means not wasting time and money looking for more.

All these treasures are pricey, but I spend far less than when I saved things up.

People die with a cache of unopened Dior at the back of the cabinet - don't let that be you. Donate all but the best. Enjoy your life and your Dior - now.

09 FAVOR STYLE OVER FASHION

*B*efore embracing chic minimalism I felt I should buy on-trend clothes each season. My closet became unaccountably overstuffed and unwieldy and I was not expecting that. Weird.

We're so assaulted by the lure of the new it's easy to forget *you don't have to live that way.* You needn't keep up with fads or gadgets or fashions. You can opt out entirely, tuning out the chatter about what's in.

Here are some ways to choose timeless style over trends.

1. Adopt a classic dress style.

Buy quality pieces that last, and suit your frame and personality, in your signature palette - whether pastels or jewel tones or black on black. Who cares what's in fashion - you wear what looks great on you.

2. Consider a stylist.

Consult an expert to help you assemble a capsule

of enduring wardrobe staples. If you currently waste money on fast fashion or 'mistakes' you never wear (we've all done it), this investment could more than pay for itself.

3. Skip the upgrade.

People feel pressure to acquire the latest phone or tablet, but we can be more conscious. I keep tech for years and only upgrade when I think it's necessary. To keep my phone looking and feeling fresh I declutter apps regularly and update the case.

4. Have a classic home style.

Opt for decor reflecting your taste and lifestyle. If buying endless homewares is a weakness, don't window shop or browse online.

5. Save time, money, and the planet.

When you opt out of trends, you never have to buy new or discard old for the sake of fashion. You feel no pressure to get the latest. You save time, money, stress, and space. And you reduce your personal load on the environment.

6. Focus on what you love.

Tune in to what you truly enjoy, and you escape the myth that some new thing will bring happiness. Has it so far? Live by your own rules, don't compare. You're free! Instead of envying others, you ponder what they're missing: clarity, simplicity, and peace.

10 RELEASE GIFTS AND MEMENTOES

I don't receive many gifts I wouldn't keep, because people know my minimalistic tendencies. Over time, this will happen for you too.

But what to do in the meantime with the *papier mâché* llama your cousin gave you last Christmas? Or the set of erotically themed guest soaps your mother thought were cute vegetable shapes?

Here's the thing. They thought of you, wanted to give you something, got it for you, took the time to wrap it. All those feelings they have for you, that's the true worth of the gift. And guess what? You've got that! That's now part of you, part of your relationship.

You don't need to keep the thing as well. The thing is a mere ticket stub. Why not let someone else enjoy the thing - and put it immediately into your donation box (we'll come to that).

Where possible, opt out of exchanging gifts and save everybody time, money and having to line up at the returns counter. Or agree to give experiences like ballet tickets or bagpipe lessons. Take each other to dinner or cocktails.

Giving is about showing each other we care. Look for non-stuff ways to express this.

The same applies to mementoes, keepsakes, children's artworks, even heirlooms. Don't hold on out of guilt. It serves the relationship far more to cherish memories, not things.

Instead of cluttering your space, you could:

1. Take photos.

Photograph the kids' creations and save them into a folder for each child. When you want to feel nostalgic, flick through your digital albums.

2. Make a memory box.

Select the items best capturing your memories and store them in a lovely box, tied up with ribbon.

3. Curate.

Choose one or two items to represent your loved one - a framed photo, a figurine they treasured - and display it as a reminder that keeps the person close.

Cherish the relationship and let the stuff go.

11 DECIDE TO DO WITHOUT

There are things we keep because we've always had them. Like that kitchen utensil everyone has but no one knows what it's for. Plus, you may need it one day to defend yourself against a spider.

Let's consider items you might relinquish.

1. Printer / Scanner.

Scanning apps let you capture documents with your phone and store them digitally. No scanner, no paper. (Of course: check whether you need physical copies of documents, and back up your files.)

As a writer I thought I'd need a printer, but I've got used to working on-screen. I no longer need to buy, monitor stocks of, and store toner, paper, and cords. When I need to print I go to my local stationery store - way better machines and lots of options. Plus for me, being around stationery is like being in nature for regular people, but with fewer bugs.

2. Seasonal decorations.

Seeing the year unfold through seasons and celebrations is joyous. (I don't get Halloween though - why *encourage* people to knock at your door?)

I only decorate for Christmas, which I celebrate secularly. I have an elegant LED tree that illuminates the corner of the living room and casts a pretty reflection on the window. It needs no decorations, a must for a lazy one such as myself - high impact, low effort, my favorite kind of minimalism. Needing no decorations saves money, storage, eventual landfill, and time. But let pleasure be your guide. If the ritual of adorning your tree charms you, then cosset your baubles and savor their joy.

3. Furniture.

Less stuff means less storage, so consider furniture you might no longer need.

- I have a set of nested small side tables to bring out as needed, so I don't require a coffee table.
- Some years ago I pulled out the few paper documents I need and stored them in small stationery drawers, recycled or shredded the rest, and donated the abomination that was my filing cabinet to blight some other poor soul's home.

- I have one beautiful, high quality set each of crockery, cutlery, napery, and glassware that's used regardless of the occasion, so I don't need a buffet or starsky or hutch for storage.

Choosing to have fewer things means less to think about, store, fall over, and bestrew the planet with. Survey your home - what could you do without?

12 DON'T BE A SQUIRREL

*S*quirrels prepare for winter by stockpiling tree bark, acorns, nuts, berries, and probably dental floss. We humans can be more relaxed with our stashes.

For efficient and chic decluttering, look for entire classes of hoarded clutter - whether furniture, books, clothes, home goods, or kitchen gadgets - to purge en masse.

Here are examples.

1. The past.

Do you have outfits for a previous career? Equipment for long-ago sports? Supplies for abandoned hobbies? Outgrown children's clothes and toys? Expired medications, condiments, skincare, cosmetics? Flip phone chargers?

Peruse your home excavating all the arcane exotica from former civilizations, check planet-friendly disposal options, and then for the love of Pete, let it go.

2. Old roles.

Many moons ago I entertained often - requiring a large dresser of plates and glasses plus the ability to spend hours at a time internally screaming. I now joyfully embrace my hermitude (not a word, but I love it) and admit my go-to dinner recipe is a cheese board, and I only occasionally have guests.

If you're of a certain age you probably recognize roles you no longer wish to play. Accepting you'll never ride through Paris in a sports car with the warm wind in your hair, you surrender the headscarves and Marianne Faithful records. Rejecting society's expectations you should be a word-class kazoo player, you donate your chests full of *Thus Spake Zarathustra* sheet music.

Let go of old roles, and with them, the expectations, pressure - and stuff.

3. One day...

Here, consider interests you thought you'd take up, projects you were going to get to, sizes you were hoping to be. Yes they may still happen, but if they've haunted your home and happiness for years, then let them go, and give yourself the kindness of buying when you're ready.

4. Spares.

It's wise to keep extras of things you use regularly - food, pharmacy items, batteries, and toiletries. But overdoing the spares causes clutter and visual stress. Plus things expire, and tastes change. Opt for an elegant amount of extras - only enough to avoid running out and save shopping time.

Also, avoid multiples when you only need one or two. Beach towels, picnic blankets, throw rugs, wine decanters, vases, storage containers, salad bowls. For some people, removing extras and doubles alone is enough to transform a dystopian hellscape into a relaxing abode.

Squirrels are cute, but living now, having only what you need, and relishing a chic minimalistic life is cuter.

13 DISCARD IMPERFECTLY

a favorite way to torture myself is to set ridiculously high standards for a goal. I agonize for ages then eventually abandon the project to avoid the inevitable failure, while sobbing quietly in the fetal position.

A slightly better approach, I have found, is to lower my expectations. Sometimes I have to keep adjusting them, lower and lower, like a psychological limbo dance, until I feel I have some shot at success.

Such was my mindset when I first desired minimalism. I felt tremendous pressure to get rid of things 'the right way'. Sell everything valuable. Donate to the ideal charities. Discard flawlessly. But what I lacked in pragmatism I also lacked in self-motivation.

In the end, I leaned into the laziness that has saved me, time and again. I chose to sell nothing, donate everything useable to one local charity (they were glad to collect the lot), and throw away the rest (I booked a refuse collection). This hugely streamlined the project.

Perhaps you are inspired to photograph, list, and sell your stuff online. Hold a yard sale. Repair things. Identify the particular charity for each class of clutter. Then you should do that.

But if you're immobilized or depressed, if this pressure is stopping you from getting rid of stuff you've had for years - or decades - then grant yourself clutter amnesty. Do the minimum and get out from under the mess.

I have donated treasures to my local thrift store - including expensive unworn clothes and fine jewelry. I viewed it as a financial donation and felt great about such a generous gift. But it was primarily a gift to myself, to be free of having to sell it.

Before you start, decide on your disposal strategy so it doesn't trip you up along the way.

1. Sell.

What, if anything, will you sell?

2. Donate.

Where will you donate? Is there a local charity collection service or drop-off?

3. Discard.

What about the detritus no one would want? Recycle what you can. Cut up things that could trap wildlife. Find out disposal rules for your area. But keep it simple!

Sometimes you have to be philosophical like Mediocrates and say, that's good enough. Next time, do better.

14 DESIGN A PLAN

S ometimes things simply work out - your personal trainer retires but a wine bar opens in the building, so you keep up your visits. Usually though, we need to plan for things to go well.

When I did my major minimalism-induced purge I listed all the spaces in my apartment, by room, on a large whiteboard. I checked each one off as I completed it. I used two vacation weeks to make a significant start and then continued on weekends. It was tiring, but it felt tinglingly good (I would open drawers and cabinets just to admire my tastefully minimalistic spaces), and I happily gave up some activities, including going out with friends and watching TV, to get it done.

How will you declutter?

1. Select a schedule.

Here are some options:

- Set aside several weekends
- Assign an hour each day
- Take a week's vacation - or two
- Complete a small area any time you feel like it - and take your time
- Set timed goals - for example: reduce the bookshelf to 50 books in 30 minutes
- Book a session with a professional organizer.

2. Create a checklist of zones.

Lists are powerful! Place yours somewhere prominent, so you can enjoy checking off completed zones and see what lies ahead. If you like schedules, allocate a time to each area. Be sure to include all that apply to your home:

- Living room
- Dining room
- Kitchen
- Bedrooms
- Bathrooms and en-suites
- Hall closets and linen presses
- Hallways
- Laundry
- Attic
- Basement
- Garage
- Shed

- Offsite storage.

3. Decide where to start.

Now you've determined *when* you'll declutter and listed *areas*, next choose *where* you'll begin. This is an important step because, as Tom Petty said, starting is the hardest part. No, wait - that was waiting. Anyway, once you're in motion, momentum will carry you along.

So where should you begin? What feels most motivating? Choose the area that's:

- Easiest to declutter
- Most fun
- Most annoying in its current state
- Somewhere you desperately want to make beautiful.

Now put it on your calendar. It's a date!

15 USE THESE THREE STEPS EVERY TIME

*H*ave you christened your storage closet *the chamber of secrets* to add intrigue to your obsolete cords and broken ab trainers? Don't worry - we're going to use a simple three-step process to deal with the stuff, no matter where it has taken up residence or how much there is. You can select a room, cabinet, cupboard, shelf, drawer, surface, whatever - the method is the same.

Ready?

Step 1. Remove everything.

Have you started yelling at me? *Isn't this unnecessary work? You're supposed to be the poster girl for lazy. Why can't I just remove the things I don't want?* You'll see why in step 3.

Step 2. Wipe it down.

This will make you feel great and your spaces will look their best too. Just a quick wipe.

Step 3. Put back ONLY the best.

In the past, I might have listed for you all the reasons to get rid of something. For instance, donate or discard clothes that don't fit well, aren't your style, feel scratchy, etc. Which meant by default, keep everything else.

Now, my approach is even more minimalistic. Don't keep something purely because there's nothing wrong with it and it ticks the boxes for functionality. You need to use *and* love it. I have a red velvet rope for my life and a threatening bouncer with upscale tastes allowing only the best in. And I suggest this for you as well. This is your one precious life. Keep only the *crème de la crème*.

As you complete step 3 for each section of your space, recall the mindset shifts we've been making. This is chic minimalism in action. Before you put *anything* back into your space:

1. Consider your values.

Does this item reflect what you care about now? Does it give you pleasure?

2. Consider the space available.

Does this item deserve a spot in the limited space you have?

3. Consider the quality.

Is this item well made? Will it last?

4. Consider simplicity.

Would you prefer simplicity to the convenience of this item?

5. Is this your best?

Do you have another version of this you love more?

I'm not suggesting you agonize over each item, rather, that you have an attitude of 'only the best'. Let these questions guide you. Perhaps the red velvet rope needs to stay in place.

16 HAVE A PLACE FOR EVERYTHING

*I*f you've looked inside my drawers - and honestly, who hasn't - you know everything has a dedicated place. It's the same in the closet, kitchen, bathroom, living area. This alignment between possessions and placement is neither sorcery nor an ability to fold things into origami swans before storage. It's three simple principles.

These guidelines help you know *where to put something* when you first find it a home. And how to *arrange* things after decluttering. And, perhaps most miraculously, where to *find things* you're looking for.

Principle 1: The more you use it, the more accessible it should be.

In the kitchen the coffee machine, kettle, and toaster can sit on the countertop, but place everything else in drawers and cabinets to keep surfaces clear and maintain a sense of order.

In the bathroom, aim for a bare vanity and store everything out of sight. Items you use daily should be closest to hand with spares and occasional medications on higher shelves.

It may seem obvious to keep everyday things handy, but many people try to keep *everything* handy, leading to visual chaos and difficulty finding anything. If you don't use it daily, put it a little further away. Even if you use it daily, keep it handy but off your surfaces.

Principle 2: Keep similar things together.

Keeping like with like gives you an instant way to decide where things should go. Got new hand weights? Don't shove them under the bed - store them with their friends, the *other* hand weights you never use (this has never happened to me). Next time you need a mini dumbbell as a paperweight, you'll know precisely where to look.

Principle 3: Store things near where you use them.

Keep things close to where they're needed - remotes in a drawer under the TV, hairdryer in a cabinet beside the power point, coffee on the shelf above the espresso machine.

Chic minimalism means uncluttered surfaces as far as the nosy eye can see (can an eye be nosy?) as well as an elegant ordering of things that aren't seen.

17 BREAK UP WITH YOUR MESS FOR GOOD

The Venn diagram of minimalists who keep old habits and those who are soon re-buried in a clutter mountain is a circle. To break up with your mess *for good*, you need new, chic minimalism habits. These small rituals keep clutter from coming back.

1. Practice OCI-OGO.

Adopt the life habit of OCI-OGO: one comes in, one goes out:

- Buy a new pair of shoes, donate an old pair
- Update your lipstick, toss an old tube
- Give the kids a new toy, ask them to give an old one away.

OCI-OGO stops you re-cluttering your home,

and you also think twice before buying anything, since the cost now includes giving up another possession. The benefits are cumulative: the more you pare down, the more precious are your remaining treasures - and the bar for buying something new gets ever higher.

2. Look after your things.

Take care of good quality belongings and you'll enjoy them for ages. Put your possessions away after use. Don't stuff things into too-small spaces. Air clothes after wearing - they'll need less washing and last beautifully. Repair things. Re-heel footwear and you'll save money and enjoy your favorites longer.

3. Perform an evening ritual.

Clear dishes. Put clothes away. Return toys and clothes to kids' rooms so they learn to care for their possessions. Place remotes in drawers, fold up rugs. Tidy surfaces and give them a wipe-down. Run a cordless vacuum over the floor (I hate housework but find this fun!). It might take twenty minutes or so, but you'll feel great and cherish your space more.

4. Establish an overflow area.

I place things 'in pending' on a dedicated shelf in a cupboard. The carton for something I may return. A gift I'm unsure about. Every month or so I go through whatever's there. Don't use this space to avoid making decisions, or let it become like Monica Gellar's secret closet. Use it as a handy area where things are allowed to be in holding - temporarily.

5. Keep things flowing out.

Cultivate a habit of looking for things that no longer deserve a place in your life. As soon as you notice - straight to the donation box.

6. Let others emulate you.

If you share a home with others, keep communal spaces as clutter-free as possible and return people's stuff to their space each evening - where they can wallow in their personal quagmires if they wish. Keep your own space minimal and beautiful and it may inspire others to follow suit. And if they ask for help, give it while letting them make their own choices.

18 SAY NO - ELEGANCE IS REFUSAL

Sometimes people and things come into your life and that's a shame. But, as Coco Chanel said, *Elegance is refusal*. A perfect mantra for chic minimalists!

A way I love to harness the elegance of saying no is to find opportunities to say a *blanket* no when making choices. This is another way laziness serves me - I love pre-made decisions! A macro-decision saves time and thought and potential mistakes, and avoids countless micro-decisions.

For example, I say a blanket no to...

1. Anything with a dominating logo.

Clothes, handbags, even stationery items. If the logo overwhelms the design, it's not for me.

2. Gifts with purchase.

It's too easy to buy things you don't need in order to qualify. Often there's a trial size of something I like in these gifts, and it's more cost-effective to buy a full size of that item and skip the rest.

3. Sales, Black Friday, etc.

If I wouldn't buy it full price, I won't buy it on sale. If something is already in my cart and goes on sale, great! Otherwise, this retail trickery wastes time and money.

4. Brands that don't make my size in clothes or footwear.

I used to order things 'in case' they fit but I've learned which brands fit me well, or well enough to need only a little tailoring. With the others, I mark their online ads irrelevant and bypass their stores, and narrow my focus to brands that cater to me.

5. Clothes stores with vast ranges.

Some stores have so many racks of packed-tight clothes, it's overwhelming. I prefer boutiques with smaller ranges, or department stores with manageable sections. Much more pleasant for my easily overloaded brain, and often better service too.

6. Superficial relationships.

Minimalism is not just about physical possessions. As an introvert I practice minimalism in my social life, cultivating deep relationships with the people I love most and saying no (pleasantly!) to casual acquaintances. This keep my engagements manageable, and feels more meaningful and satisfying too.

7. Organized activities.

I cherish my relationships and prioritize being a good friend. But I draw the line at organized activities. This allows an easy macro-decision about baby showers and other such ordeals.

Where can you apply the elegance of refusal, and say a once-and-for-all no?

Decide to minimize decisions. It brings a lovely feeling of serenity and white space to your life.

19 CULTIVATE A DONATION HABIT

There's a curious bond that can form between a girl and the lame miscellanea she orders when trying to avoid her feelings. But we can break that bond by having a permanent, easily accessible donation box. Anything can go in there - no guilt, no questions asked.

Here are some ideas.

1. Make your donation receptacle beautiful.

Repurpose a box in which you received something lovely, or a large robust bag, or allocate a drawer or shelf. Make it substantial enough to accommodate many things and pretty enough to make you feel good when you look at it.

2. Put it in a convenient location where you see it often.

Somewhere near the door is great. I have a shelf on a credenza where I can place things without their looking untidy, but which offers an automatic reminder to drop them off when I pop out for errands.

3. Choose your charity.

Know in advance where your donations will go so there's no friction between thinking you'd like to let something go and getting it to someone who can use it. I have a thrift store on my way to the local shops, making it a simple fortnightly task (I batch and complete errands every two weeks) to hand over whatever has piled up. You may prefer to find somewhere on a regular driving route.

4. Think of expensive items as monetary donations.

Recently I bought a designer top that was super chic and fitted like it was made for me. But although I put it on many times before going out, it was cumbersome and I invariably ended up wearing something else. We've all made these big-budget blunders and felt we can't just throw away something pricey.

As I've mentioned, I made my peace with giving away costly mistakes by thinking of them as financial donations: would I be happy to donate that much money to the charity? *Bien sûr!* If you have expensive things that feel 'too good' to give away, think of them as a wad of cash and happily hand them over.

20 DON'T RESIST TEMPTATION

*O*scar Wilde said, *I can resist anything except temptation*, and those of us who like nice things can relate. Maybe your minimalism goal was to declutter 100 things. Only 200 to go!

As chic minimalists, how do we deal with tantalizing online ads and offers? Impulse buys at the store? The add-to-cart allure when our defenses are down after we've had a glass or two?

Here are some strategies.

1. Unsubscribe.

Detach from the influx of *what's new* and *great offers*. Unfollow, unsubscribe, install ad blockers. You can't avoid it all when you're online, but you can reduce the onslaught.

2. Slow your scroll.

Don't scroll social media when you're tired, upset, or tipsy. All the pretty things will still be there tomorrow when you're better equipped to take good care of yourself and choose wisely.

3. Decide in advance what you'll let go.

When you're considering a purchase, remember OCI-OGO. Develop a habit of asking what you'll release in order to buy this. Perhaps this item is exceptional quality, aligned with your values, and better than something else you'll donate. That sounds like a good purchase. If not, turn it down.

4. Say a hard no to cheapie sites and stores.

You know the ones. They sell disposable rubbish that hurts the environment, your good taste, and possibly the people employed to make them. Cut them off at the pass - walk away, unfollow, unsubscribe, click the option that says the ad is not right for you. Don't start a relationship with them and if you're in one, get out of it - and close the door behind you.

No matter how effective our decluttering, we'll revert to excess if we keep buying more. Be strategic and, where possible, cut off temptation before it gets to you.

21 SHOP STRATEGICALLY

*W*hat if you genuinely need something? An outfit for a special occasion. A tranquilizer dart for the neighbor's kid who just took up the recorder. How does a chic minimalist navigate the lure of stores and sites that use cunning psychological warfare to make us buy more than we need?

Try these tips.

1. Keep your values in mind.

A fun idea is to choose three words reflecting your values and let these guide your purchases. For instance my current words when buying clothes are *elegant*, *relaxed*, (a little bit) *sexy*. I already have good basics, and I've learned I won't wear anything remotely fussy, no matter how gorgeous, so these words orient me to focus on the gaps in my closet.

For homewares my words are *modern, sleek, neutral.* Choosing values-related keywords can help you match your style and avoid those dreaded *it-was-on-sale!* errors.

2. Take a cooling-off period.

If you spot something you want, give yourself breathing room. At a physical store I ask if they can hold the item for half an hour, and I do other shopping. Online I add to cart and do something else. Stepping away lets you take a break and avoid impulsive buys.

3. Choose returns-friendly online stores.

Check returns policies and favor stores that make it super easy to return things.

When a purchase arrives, inspect it, test it, try it on, and decide *at once* if you're keeping it. If it's ideal, put it away and recycle the packaging. If you don't love it - if it's okay or kinda looks fine - package it up for return *now*, and place it by the door to take to the post office or store. Save the money for something you adore and avoid the clutter.

4. Have a red velvet rope for your life.

As a chic minimalist, you have high standards and are careful what you let into your life. Remember - there's a bouncer keeping all the riff-raff out and only lifting the rope for those few things that align with your values, give you pleasure, are excellent quality, and are worth your space, time, and money.

. . .

Be the editor of your home and your life. Curate the best, take care of your possessions, derive pleasure from them, and only buy what you love.

Congratulations - you are a chic minimalist!

MERCI

*T*hank you for reading *Chic Minimalism: 21 Rules For Mastering The Art Of Less*.

Embracing less has brought me peace, pleasure, and a much more meaningful life - so I'm thrilled to share my little rules with you. I sincerely hope you find the joys of chic minimalism in your own life.

If you would like to hear about future books in my *Quick Read* series, please subscribe to my free, irregular, and delightful dispatches. I'll be sending you samples of new books - so you can enjoy a little taster of many exciting topics to come.

Sign up micheleconnolly.com.

If you liked this book, I would be so very grateful if you would share a quick review on Amazon. Reviews are *everything* to an author. Plus, they are such a help to other readers. So, thank you.

Till next time,

Au revoir,

Michele

ABOUT THE AUTHOR

Michele Connolly is an introvert, minimalist, award-winning author, and misfit. She is known for her honest, succinct, and humorous writing style.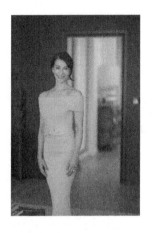

After leaving a corporate career, Michele gained a bachelor of psychology, wrote a first class honors thesis on personality and happiness, became a certified life coach, and discovered cronuts, so it was a significant time.

Her books, programs, and websites have helped tens of thousands of people around the world to enjoy being an introvert, declutter, get organized, and simplify life.

To stay in touch, follow Michele online or sign up for her updates at micheleconnolly.com.

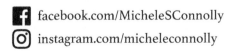

facebook.com/MicheleSConnolly

instagram.com/micheleconnolly

Made in United States
North Haven, CT
07 March 2024

49605599R00046